Heads Up! Self-Defense For Journalists

By Randal Seyler

Featuring essays by the
Art of Manliness creators
Brett and Kate McKay
(www.artofmanliness.com)

Heads Up! Self-Defense For Journalists

ISBN 978-0-359-50746-7

DEDICATION

This is a book about self-defense, meant for journalists and other media personnel, but the information contained applies to everyone.

My experience as a journalist, human resources professional, and longtime karate student and teacher, made me want to write an article or Powerpoint presentation for the Arkansas Press Association on personal safety for media professionals.

I started on this project in October 2017 following the Las Vegas shooting that claimed 58 lives at a country music concert. As I finish up the book, a gunman in New Zealand has just killed at least 50 people who were attending mosque.

You'll notice there aren't any punches or kicks in this book. That's because they are pretty much useless against a machine gun. Once the bullets start to fly, run like hell away from the shooting.

The best defense is to be aware of your surroundings, have a plan of what to do if you are at work or out in the public and a terror attack begins.

If you only take away one thought from this book, let it be this: Be aware of your surroundings. That requires using the best self-defense tool you have: Your brain.

I want to dedicate this book to my wife, **Shannon,** and my numerous martial arts instructors and peers, in particular, the late **Walter Burmick Appleby** sensei of Dumas, Arkansas, who introduced me to Taiho-Ryu Karate and taught me the difference between puppies and tigers.

INTRODUCTION

I started work on this project the night after the Oct. 1, 2017, shooting in Las Vegas claimed 58 lives and injured 851 people.

I am writing this introduction just eight months later, the day after a shooter killed five newspaper employees in Annapolis, Maryland.

My initial plan for this project was a Powerpoint presentation for journalists, one that could be shared with press associations and newspapers so they could pass on the information and maybe help keep some people alive when a worst case scenario happens.

According to the website, theguardian.com, there were 101 mass shootings between Oct. 1, 2017, and Feb. 15, 2018 which was the day a deranged ex-student walked into the Marjory Stoneman Douglas High School in Parkland, Florida, leaving 17 bodies and 17 wounded in his wake.

In roughly a three-fourths of a year, somewhere around 2,000 people had died in mass shootings.

Add to that a president who calls the media "the enemy of the American people" (New York Times, Feb. 17, 2017) and a National Rifle Association spokesperson who threatens the media that "their time is up" (USA Today, March 5, 2018), and the need for a media safety training program becomes obvious.

Reporters are not only targets in their workplaces, they also are often at the scene of violent episodes, are plainly visible in public forums, and often write about crime and criminals, who can become disgruntled, as early reports seem to indicate was the case in Annapolis.

Awareness is the best self-defense tool we have, and as reporters, we should be more aware than the average person because our job is to see details that others miss.

Hopefully this book will help you become more aware of your own safety.

CHAPTER ONE

It was nearly 20 years ago that I had my first serious brush with workplace violence.

I was working in human resources in a large manufacturing plant in Fayetteville, Arkansas, where I was the HR coordinator for the second and third shifts, which meant I worked 3 p.m. to midnight.

As part of my job, I was also the person responsible for the safety and security departments once the plant's safety manager had gone home.

One summer evening, around 7 p.m., I got a call that an unauthorized person was seen within the plant, but the intruder was now no where to be found. I met with the lead security guard and the evening plant manager and, after a brief discussion, we split up and went in search of our intruder.

The three of us each had about 100,000 square feet of factory to search.

After about 30 minutes of playing hide-and-seek, I received a radio call saying to come to the paint room, an employee had been assaulted.

To make a long story short, the employee was punched in the face by a jealous neighbor who thought the employee was too friendly with his wife. The neighbor knew where and when the employee worked, so he snuck into the plant, found the employee, beat him up, then fled.

Obviously, plant security was not very stringent — the facility manufactured aluminum wheels and had a foundry for melting the metal, so in the humid Arkansas summers, every door of the building stood wide open all night long.

There was no perimeter fence, except for a wooden privacy fence that enclosed the outside break area. Luckily for the employee, and all his co-workers (including me), disgruntled neighbor was only punch-happy, not murderous. All he got for his alleged indiscretions were a black eye and a bloody nose.

If the neighbor had walked into the plant with an assault rifle, the results could have been horrific.

Now, nearly two decades on, the United States has been literally awash in the blood of innocent victims of insane violence — not only in workplaces, but in schools, shopping malls, and even at concerts. The 2017 Las Vegas massacre should have been a wake-up call to the nation, but politics and ignorance —and ignorant politicians — did nothing to make the streets safer.

But that's OK. The first lesson of this book is this axiom:

You are responsible for your safety.

No matter where you are, and no matter who might be legally responsible for your personal well being, ultimately, it's what you do in times of crisis that can mean the difference between life and death. The most important of these things is stay alert to your environment (thus the title — Heads Up!)

There are things you can do to keep safe, and teaching you those safety tips is the purpose of this book.

CHAPTER TWO

I'm a long-time karate practitioner and instructor.

I have been enamored of the Asian martial arts since I was a teen, watching the movie "Billy Jack" for the first time in a theater at the age of 12 or so, then watching "Kung Fu" on ABC each week set me on a course of discovery and learning that even today, nearly half a century later, I still enjoy.

Over the years I have studied half a dozen different karate, tae kwon do and kung fu styles, and I also was inspired to study a variety of topics, from philosophy and religion to physical fitness and nutrition.

As a martial artist and as a karate teacher, I found myself studying business and organization and even education theory and teaching skills.

It's hard to really put a label on what martial arts has meant to me. To me, "karate guy" is my first self-definition. My second self-definition would be journalist, which has been my profession for over three decades.

There was a 15-year period in the middle of my journalism career where I wound up working in the manufacturing industry by happenstance, and during which I worked on the side as a freelance writer as well as editor of a few literary magazines.

During my manufacturing industry career, I not only received valuable management experience, I also got my first-hand experiences with workplace security and safety, and that was really the motivation that set me thinking about how to apply my (then two decades of karate experience) to workplace safety.

I also had my four years of military experience in there where I had met a variety of safety concerns and survived them — most of which involved drunken rows with fellow sailors and Marines, as well as various karate skirmishes in practice and in competition.

Typically books about surviving violence are written by authors with either police experience or military experience. Both of those perspectives are valuable, especially to fellow police and military professionals.

But I want to approach the topic from the innocent bystander perspective.

You've probably heard of the kung fu animals — tiger, snake, dragon, crane, panther. If innocent bystanders had a "kung fu animal," it would probably be the rabbit, and that's the animal we want to imitate out in the field (or even out for the evening with friends).

Alert, fleet of foot, and ready to bolt at the first sign of a hawk — that's how I want you to be.

Also, most manuals on survival are written either in a past-tense mode — as in, these people should have done A, B, and C to survive — or they are written sort of depressingly, so much so that I hear the voice of Eeyore in my head when I read them. The gist of the text is "it's all going to end in tears."

In Hollywood, Karate Guy TM jumps into the biker bar full of toughs twice his side, all armed to the teeth, and Karate Guy TM makes quick work of them all with feet and fists a-flailing.

That scenario is a fantasy that has nothing at all to do with either karate or reality.

Ultimately, the highest skill is the ability to sense violence brewing and either avoid the situation or, if necessary, de-escalate the situation.

However, having some self-defense training is always useful. Many police departments will offer free self-defense classes, and most towns have karate, taekwondo or jujitsu schools. Krav Maga is a particularly effective, no-nonsense self-defense art.

Fitness also is important. Be as fit as you can be, and exercise regularly — running, jogging or at least fast walking is important. If you have physical limitations, you should obviously take them into account, but be as fit as possible.

The best way to not be hit is to not get into a fight, and the best way to not get shot is to not be where people are shooting at you. In either case, the ability to flee is of utmost importance.

CHAPTER THREE

Personally, I have had a few encounters with violence, mostly minor — except for being relieved at gunpoint in San Diego of my empty wallet, and I escaped that incident unscathed by running like a rabbit while being shot at.

One of the modern pioneers of karate, Iain Abernathy, has written one of the best explanations of the idea of true self-defense, versus the "Walker, Texas Ranger" fantasy of karate making one capable of defeating rooms full of villains, or the Charles Atlas "90-pound weakling" fantasy of martial arts as vengeance for social slight.

"True civilian self-protection should focus on the skills needed to avoid, escape and defuse situations. It should be in accordance with the law of the land and include what to do after the event. If physical action is required, then the last thing we want is a 'fight.'" Abernathy writes.

"When it comes to the physical side of self-protection, we don't aim to 'fight to win' but to fight to escape and to fight to keep ourselves safe. We don't need to 'win' the fight. What we need to do to truly 'win' is to entirely avoid anything that even resembles a fight."

Thinking self-protection and street fighting are one and the same is dangerous thinking which can lead to dangerous practice, Abernathy warns. "Approaching self-protection with a fighting methodology runs counter to the objective and is likely to lead to a failure to avoid conflict, physical harm and legal difficulties."

What this means is you don't have to have the karate skills of a wizened master, or the fighting ability of a Navy SEAL to stay safe — you just have to be able to think like a warrior and keep an open mind when it comes to thinking about your own personal safety, and the safety of your loved ones.

There is a difference between prepared and paranoid, and sometimes that division seems razor thin. The ability to listen to your instinct when you think something may be wrong, and seeing danger in every possible scenario, can become a slippery slope — especially for survivors of violent attacks who may be dealing with Post Traumatic Stress Syndrome on top of feelings of fear and guilt.

If you have survived a life-threatening event, counseling is often the best way to overcome your emotional turmoil. But keep in mind that lightning may strike twice, and just because you survived one bad thing doesn't mean another bad thing can't be hiding in your future.

That may sound harsh, or even paranoid, but take into account your personal and professional circumstances.

You may work as a bank teller and only be violently assaulted and robbed once in your career – but if you are a convenience store clerk, the possibility of violent assault is a day-to-day threat, and you could be robbed numerous times in a career.

A similar comparison could be made between police officers and emergency medical technicians. Both professionals respond to violence scenes, but the chances of a violent encounter are greater for the policeman than the EMT, although both groups of professionals often find themselves in dangerous situations.

Even within the military, there are certain classifications of soldiers, such as Green Berets, Delta Force, or Infantry who are much more likely to find themselves in harm's way than other groups, such as supply clerks or administrators.

The ability to recognize and assess threat levels within your own circumstances is vital to your well being.

CHAPTER FOUR

In some countries, being a journalist is a dangerous profession.

Mexico and Russia are two places currently where being a reporter can be hazardous to your health.

Wikipedia lists 180 dead journalists in Mexico between January 2007 and December 2017, not including Gumaro Pérez Aguilando, a Mexican journalist has been shot dead while he attended his son's school Christmas pageant as attacks on the country's press continue unabated. Aguilando was killed on Dec. 19, 2017.

In Russia, Wikipedia lists 140 dead journalists since 2000, all falling under the reign of President Valdimir Putin.

By contrast, in the U.S. Wikipedia lists only 5 journalists killed since 2000 for pursuing their careers. However, 6 media workers and 1 non-working journalist died in the Sept. 11, 2001, terror attacks — which would bring the total to 12.

One working photojournalist, Bill Biggart, who was killed by falling debris as he was taking photographs of the New York City Twin Towers.

According to the website www.statista.com, which features statistics and studies from more than 18,000 sources, 780 journalists worldwide were killed between 2007 and 2017.

For perspective, in the U.S. alone, 1,672 police officers were killed between 2006 and 2016, according to the National Law Enforcement Officers Memorial Fund website, www.nleomf.org.

A convenience store clerk's job can be even more dangerous than a police officer's, according to the U.S. Department of Labor's Bureau of Labor Statistics.

The agency found 52 convenience store employees were killed in 2009, compared to the 46 officers who were slain that year, the Athens Banner-Herald reported in 2011.

CHAPTER FIVE

What about gun-toting civilians saving the day?

Dr. Paige Schilt, writing for garnetnews.com, recalled a workplace violence episode at University of Texas in Austin and the reactions of students. Schilt is the interim director of the Sanger Learning Center at the University of Texas at Austin and the author of "Queer Rock Love: A Family Memoir."

"I looked out that same window on May 1 of last year, but from a different vantage point. On that day, I was huddled under my desk, hoping to see what was happening below without getting hit by a stray bullet. One of my co-workers had run into the building, yelling for students to get inside offices or classrooms and hide. I assumed that there was an active shooter, and I prayed that my wooden door—the same kind of door that encloses thousands of dorm rooms—would be thick enough to stop a bullet.

As it turns out, there was no campus shooter. My quick-thinking colleague was shepherding people inside because a student suffering from mental health issues was attacking people with a hunting knife on the plaza between the dorm and the gym. One student was killed and three others were wounded before police apprehended the suspect on the steps of our building.

"As tragic as that day was, it could easily have become much, much worse. You see, the state of Texas allows concealed firearms on public campuses. If the police hadn't apprehended the alleged assailant so quickly, there's evidence to suggest that an armed civilian might have attempted to intervene.

"Moments after campus authorities issued an "all clear" message, one of my coworkers spoke to a student who claimed that he had been en route to grab his gun, which was stored nearby. Another colleague was visited in her office by a former student from one of her classes. He alluded to his concealed handgun and promised to "protect" her if anything like this happened again.

"I understand the impulse to arm students with every protection within our grasp. However, as a parent and an educator, I look to experts to help me evaluate which interventions will truly help keep my own and other children safe.

"In a 2008 survey of university police chiefs, an overwhelming 86% of the chiefs disagreed or strongly disagreed with the proposition that concealed carry would prevent campus killings. More recently, public health researchers at Johns Hopkins University analyzed data from 2009-2015 and found that, "successful civilian uses of guns to stop a mass shooting were incredibly rare and about as common as armed civilians being shot while attempting to respond to mass shooting incidents."

Why are successful civilian interventions in mass shootings so rare?

The authors of the Johns Hopkins report concluded that "shooting accurately and making appropriate judgments about when and how to shoot in chaotic, high-stress situations" requires skills and tactical training that the average concealed-carry permit holder simply doesn't have.

"My own experience with the stabbing incident last May indicates just how unlikely it is that untrained civilians will make appropriate, unbiased judgments in a chaotic, high-stress situation. Because the fatal victim was white and the alleged perpetrator was black, the incident triggered a kind of racial panic on campus. Before I had even crawled out from under my desk, I saw rumors on social media that the violence was part of a coordinated attack on frat houses and other predominantly white residential enclaves.

"It may be tempting to think that this vigilantism is just a Texas problem. But in fact, the NRA has been pushing a nationwide program of campus carry legislation ever since the Virginia Tech shooting in 2007. Since that time, bills that would force colleges to allow guns on campus have been introduced in 20 different states. In 2015, Texas became the eighth state to pass such a law.

Arkansas, my home state, passed a similar law in 2017. A gun is only as good as the person wielding it, and for the most part, that is a pretty low bar. On the website, artofmanliness.com, Brett and Kate McKay explain why the average person isn't really ready to stage a firefight with an armed perpetrator.

"If you're like most Americans, you're probably overweight and out of shape. Sure, there are some health consequences that can make life complicated and expensive, but for the most part, being overweight and out of shape isn't much of a problem in our cushy world," the McKays write.

"But when the SHTF, that spare tire around your waist can prevent you from saving your life or the lives of those around you. The strain that that extra weight causes on your body can quickly put you out of commission or make you utterly useless from the get-go.

"At the gun class I go to at the United States Shooting Academy, about 70% of the students are obese. I'm talking candidate-for-gastric-bypass surgery obese. When we were doing drills on firing from behind cover, the instructor had us alternating from a kneeling position to a standing position. Two of the guys in our group couldn't do it at all and many were breathing heavily from the simple exercise.
"At a smaller class consisting of mostly in-shape guys, the instructor brought up the fact that a lot of people coming through the academy were really out of shape. "They think because they have a gun, they don't need to run or kneel or crouch," he said. "What they don't realize is not every fight is a gun fight and if you truly want to be effective as a fighter, you've got to be in shape physically, if only for the stress management advantage it gives you."

"Toting around a weapon, even if you're skilled in using it, doesn't automatically make a man a sheepdog. If you don't have the physical and mental fitness to thrive in a variety of situations, you're just a sheep with a Glock.

CHAPTER SIX

Some facts about active shooter incidents.

The FBI studied active shooter situations in 2014 to try and make some sense out of the phenomena.

The agreed-upon definition of an active shooter by U.S. government agencies—including the White House, U.S. Department of Justice/FBI, U.S. Department of Education, and U.S. Department of Homeland Security/ Federal Emergency Management Agency — is "an individual actively engaged in killing or attempting to kill people in a confined and populated area."3 Implicit in this definition is that the subject's criminal actions involve the use of firearms.4 For purposes of its study, the FBI extended this definition to include individuals, because some incidents involved two or more shooters.

Though the federal definition includes the word "confined," the FBI excluded this word in its study, as the term confined could omit incidents that occurred outside a building.
As a result, the FBI identified 160 active shooter incidents that occurred in the United States between 2000 and 2013.8

Although additional active shooter incidents may have occurred during this time period, the FBI is confident this research captured the vast majority of incidents falling within the search criteria.

Of that 160 incidents, 1,043 casualties including 486 killed and 557 wounded – that's an average of 11.4 incidents a year, with an increasing trend from 2000 to 2013, according to the FBI study.

 Other facts revealed:

• An average of 6.4 incidents occurred in the first 7 years studied, and an average of 16.4 occurred in the last 7 years.

• 70 percent of the incidents occurred in either a commerce/business or educational environment.

• Shootings occurred in 40 of 50 states and the District of Columbia.

• 60 percent of the incidents ended before police arrived.

Casualties

• Casualties (victims killed and wounded) totaled 1,043. The individual shooters are not included in this total.

• A total of 486 individuals were killed.

• A total of 557 individuals were wounded.

• In 64 incidents (40.0 percent), the crime would have fallen within the federal definition of "mass killing"—defined as "three or more" killed—under the new federal statute.

Incidents with highest casualty counts

• Cinemark Century 16 Theater in Aurora, Colorado: 70 (12 killed, 58 wounded), July 20, 2012.

• Virginia Polytechnic Institute and State University in Blacksburg, Virginia: 49 (32 killed, 17 wounded), April 16, 2007.12

• Ft. Hood Soldier Readiness Processing Center in Ft. Hood, Texas: 45 (13 killed, 32 wounded), November 5, 2009.

• Sandy Hook Elementary School and a residence in Newtown, Connecticut: 29 (27 killed, 2 wounded), December 14, 2012.

Shooters

• All but 2 incidents involved a single shooter.

• In at least 9 incidents, the shooter first shot and killed a family member(s) in a residence before moving to a more public location to continue shooting.

• In at least 6 incidents, the shooters were female.

• In 64 incidents (40.0 percent), the shooters committed suicide; 54 shooters did so at the scene of the crime. • At least 5 shooters from 4 incidents remain at large.

Findings

In this study, the FBI identified 160 active shooter incidents, noting they occurred in small and large towns, in urban and rural areas, and in 40 of 50 states and the District of Columbia.

Though incidents occurred primarily in commerce and educational environments (70.0 percent), they also occurred on city streets, on military and other government properties, and in private residences, health care facilities, and houses of worship. The shooters victimized young and old, male and female, family members, and people of all races, cultures, and religions.

The findings establish an increasing frequency of incidents annually. During the first 7 years included in the study, an average of 6.4 incidents occurred annually. In the last 7 years of the study, that average increased to 16.4 incidents annually. This trend reinforces the need to remain vigilant regarding prevention efforts and for law enforcement to aggressively train to better respond to—and help communities recover from—active shooter incidents.

The findings also reflect the damage that can occur in a matter of minutes. In 63 incidents where the duration of the incident could be ascertained, 44 (69.8 percent) of 63 incidents ended in 5 minutes or less, with 23 ending in 2 minutes or less. Even when law enforcement was present or able to respond within minutes, civilians often had to make life and death decisions, and, therefore, should be engaged in training and discussions on decisions they may face.

Resolutions

The majority of the 160 incidents (90, or 56.3 percent) ended on the shooter's initiative— sometimes when the shooter committed suicide or stopped shooting, and other times when the shooter fled the scene.

There were at least 25 incidents where the shooter fled the scene before police arrived. In 4 additional incidents, at least 5 shooters fled the scene and were still at large at the time the study results were released.

In other incidents, it was a combination of actions by citizens and/or law enforcement that ended the shootings. In at least 65 (40.6 percemt) of the 160 incidents, citizen engagement or the shooter committing suicide ended the shooting at the scene before law enforcement arrived. Of those:

• In 37 incidents (23.1 percent), the shooter committed suicide at the scene before police arrived.

• In 21 incidents (13.1 percent), the situation ended after unarmed citizens safely and successfully restrained the shooter. In 2 of those incidents, off-duty law enforcement officers were present and assisted.

• Of note, 11 of the incidents involved unarmed principals, teachers, other school staff and students who confronted shooters to end the threat (9 of those shooters were students).

• In 5 incidents (3.1 percent), the shooting ended after armed individuals who were not law enforcement personnel exchanged gunfire with the shooters. In these incidents, 3 shooters were killed, 1 was wounded, and 1 committed suicide.

• The individuals involved in these shootings included a citizen with a valid firearms permit and armed security guards at a church, an airline counter, a federally managed museum, and a school board meeting.

• In 2 incidents (1.3 percent), 2 armed, off-duty police officers engaged the shooters, resulting in the death of the shooters. In 1 of those incidents, the off-duty officer assisted a responding officer to end the threat.

Even when law enforcement arrived quickly, many times the shooter still chose to end his life.

In 17 (10.6 percent) of the 160 incidents, the shooter committed suicide at the scene after law enforcement arrived but before officers could act. In 45 (28.1 percent) of the 160 incidents, law enforcement and the shooter exchanged gunfire. Of those 45 incidents, the shooter was killed at the scene in 21, killed at another location in 4, wounded in 9, committed suicide in 9, and surrendered in 2.

CHAPTER SEVEN

How to Master the OODA Loop

(Editor's note) This chapter is the essay, "The Tao of Boyd: How to Master the OODA Loop," written by Brett and Kate McKay, and published on the website artofmanliness.com. It is used with permission of the authors, and includes some incredibly helpful thoughts on crisis management.

John Boyd is described by some as the greatest military strategist in history that no one knows. He began his military career as a fighter pilot in the Korean War, but he slowly transformed himself into one of the greatest philosopher-warriors to ever live.

In 1961, at age 33, he wrote "Aerial Attack Study," which codified the best dogfighting tactics for the first time, became the "bible of air combat," and revolutionized the methods of every air force in the world.

His Energy-Maneuverability (E-M) Theory helped give birth to the legendary F-15, F-16, and A-10 aircraft.

Perhaps his most significant contribution to military strategy, though, came from a series of briefings he gave. In them, Boyd laid out a way of thinking about conflict that would revolutionize warfare around the world.

The idea centers on an incredible strategic tool: the OODA Loop — Observe, Orient, Decide, Act. Nation-states around the world and even terrorist organizations use the OODA Loop as part of their military strategy. It has also been adopted by businesses to help them thrive in a volatile and highly competitive economy.

The OODA Loop is an oft-cited, but typically misunderstood idea. If you've heard of it, it was most likely presented in a fairly superficial way – as a 4-step decision-making process where the individual or group who makes it through all the stages the quickest, wins. That's one element of the OODA Loop, but there's much more to it than that.

The reason the OODA Loop is so frequently misunderstood is that John Boyd never described it in detail in a technical paper. In fact, despite all his contributions to military strategy, he only has one very short paper to his name – "Destruction and Creation." Instead, he developed and explained the OODA Loop through a series of sometimes five-hour-long briefings. The only notes we have are his briefing slides and a few tape recordings and transcripts that exist of his presentations. (Because he never wrote his ideas down, militaries and businesses often use his ideas without giving him credit. The lack of documentation likely explains why so few people today know about John Boyd.)

As you look through these materials, you quickly learn that a lot of hard thinking and philosophizing went into the development of the OODA Loop. Boyd combined a deep understanding of military history and strategic thinking with a wide range of other intellectual domains and theorems, including quantum mechanics, cybernetics, chaos theory, Popperism, and Neo-Darwinism. For this reason, to truly understand the OODA Loop, one must be familiar with the scientific and philosophical developments that helped create it.

Thus, once you move past the simplified, Cliff Notes version of the OODA Loop, you find that it's actually pretty heady stuff. It's not "groundbreaking" in the sense of revealing insight never before conceived; rather, its power is in the way it makes explicit, that which is usually implicit. It takes the basic ways we think, decide, and operate in the world — ways that often get confused and jumbled in the face of conflict and confusion — and codifies and organizes them into a strategic, effective system that can allow you to thrive in the heat of battle. It is a learning system, a method for dealing with uncertainty, and a strategy for winning head-to-head contests and competitions. In war, business, or life, the OODA Loop can help you grapple with changing, challenging circumstances and come out the other side on top.

I have spent the last month diving deep into the OODA Loop – reading everything available on it, from Boyd's briefing notes to biographies to analyses of the theory by other authors. I also met with Curtis Sprague, a former U.S. Air Marshal and Lead Instructor at the Federal Air Marshal School in Dallas, and an avid student and instructor of the OODA Loop, to get his insights. Below you will find a synthesis of what I have learned. My goal is to provide the most thorough, but also accessible primer on the OODA Loop out there. To begin your journey in mastering the "Tao of Boyd," read on.

Why We Live in Uncertainty

"Ambiguity is central to Boyd's vision... not something to be feared but something that is a given... We never have complete and perfect information. The best way to succeed is to revel in ambiguity." – Grant Hammond, *"The Mind of War: John Boyd and American Security"*

According to Boyd, ambiguity and uncertainty surround us. While the randomness of the outside world plays a large role in that uncertainty, Boyd argues that our inability to properly make sense of our changing reality is the bigger hindrance.

When our circumstances change, we often fail to shift our perspective and instead continue to try to see the world as we feel it should be. We need to shift what Boyd calls our existing "mental concepts" – or what I like to call "mental models" – in order to deal with the new reality.

Mental models – or paradigms – are simply a way of looking at and understanding the world. They create our expectations for how the world works. They are sometimes culturally relative and can be rooted in tradition, heritage, and even genetics. They can be something as specific as traffic laws or social etiquette. Or they can be as general as the overarching principles of an organization or a field of study like psychology, history, the laws and theories of science and math, and military doctrines on the rules of engagement. Because Boyd was more interested in using the OODA Loop as an organizing principle for a grand strategy, he tended to focus on these more abstract types of mental models.

While our paradigms work and match up with reality most of the time, sometimes they don't. Sometimes the universe pitches us a curveball that we never saw coming and the mental models we have to work with aren't really useful. If someone runs a red light, or kisses us in greeting instead of shaking our hand, we are surprised and momentarily thrown off our game. If an archaeologist were to uncover evidence that humans rode around on dinosaurs, previous theories on the earth's history would be thrown into disarray.

Boyd points to three philosophical and scientific principles to show that trying to understand a randomly changing universe with pre-existing mental models only results in confusion, ambiguity, and more uncertainty. Understanding the basics of these principles helps to show how uncertainty and ambiguity are not just errors in human understanding or logic, but are truly built into the framework of the universe – both the worlds outside and inside ourselves. Those three principles are Gödel's Proof, Heisenberg's Uncertainty Principle, and the 2nd Law of Thermodynamics:

Gödel's Incompleteness Theorems.
Boyd inferred from Gödel's Incompleteness Theorems that any logical model of reality is incomplete (and

possibly inconsistent) and must be continuously refined/ adapted in the face of new observations.

However, as our observations about the world become more and more precise and subtle, a second principle kicks in which limits our ability to observe reality correctly: Heisenberg's Uncertainty Principle.

Heisenberg's Uncertainty Principle.

In a nutshell, this principle shows that we cannot simultaneously fix or determine the velocity and position of a particle or body. We can measure coordinates or movements of those particles, but not both. As we get a more and more precise measure of one value (velocity or positions), our measurement of the other value becomes more and more uncertain. The uncertainty of one variable is created simply by the act of observation.

Applying this principle to understanding the world around us, Boyd inferred that even as we get more precise observations about a particular domain, we're likely to experience more uncertainty about another. Hence, there is a limitation in our ability to observe reality with precision.

Take the case of Kodak. Even though the company invented the core technology used in digital cameras today, they were so focused on traditional film that they failed to see that the emerging trend towards digital would ultimately consume the photo industry. By holding to their mental model that traditional film would always be around, they missed the fact that the landscape was rapidly shifting around them, eventually leading to the storied company having to file for bankruptcy.

2nd Law of Thermodynamics

Applying the Second Law of Thermodynamics to understanding reality, Boyd infers that individuals or organizations that don't communicate with the outside world by getting new information about the environment or by creating new mental models act like a "closed system." And just as a closed system in nature will have increasing entropy, or disorder, so too will a person or organization experience mental entropy or disorder if they're cut off from the outside world and new information.

The more we rely on outdated mental models even while the world around us is changing, the more our mental "entropy" goes up.

Think of an army platoon that's been cut off from communication with the rest of the regiment. The isolated platoon likely has an idea, or mental model, of where the enemy is located and their capabilities, but things have changed since they last talked to command. As they continue to work with their outdated mental model against a changing reality, confusion, disorder, and frustration are the results.

Boyd took insights from Gödel's Theorems, Heisenberg's Uncertainty Principle, and the Second Law of Thermodynamics and synthesized them into his own principle for what happens when we try to force old mental models onto new circumstances:

"Taken together, these three notions support the idea that any inward-oriented and continued effort to improve the match concept with observed reality will only increase the degree of mismatch."

The crux of Boyd's case for why uncertainty abounds is that individuals and organizations often look inward and apply familiar mental models that have worked in the past to try to solve new problems. When these old mental models don't work, they will often keep trying to make them work — maybe if they just use an old strategy with more gusto, things will pan out. But they don't. Business magnate Charlie Munger calls this tendency to use the familiar even in the face of a changing reality the "man with a hammer syndrome." You know the old saying: "to the man with only a hammer, everything is a nail." So it is with folks with one or two mental models to work with. Every problem can be solved with their current way of thinking. And so they keep hammering away, confused and disillusioned that their work isn't producing any results.
These folks never stop to ask, "Maybe I need a different tool?"

The Tao of Boyd: The OODA Loop

"It is a state of mind, a learning of the oneness of things, an appreciation for fundamental insights known in Eastern philosophy and religion as simply the Way [or Tao]. For Boyd, the Way is not an end but a process, a journey...The connections, the insights that flow from examining the world in different ways, from different perspectives, from routinely examining the opposite proposition, were what were important. The key is mental agility." – *Grant Hammond*

So how do we overcome this uncertainty or mental entropy? It was a question that John Boyd spent his entire life (up until the day he died) trying to answer. The OODA Loop was the result.

To the uninitiated, Boyd's full vision of the OODA Loop can look like a bunch of gobbledygook. But once you understand the thinking and philosophizing that went into creating this paradigm, you'll soon realize how incredibly insightful and profound it is.

Below, I take you on a deep journey through John Boyd's OODA Loop. My goal is to show you that it isn't merely the simple four-step decision-making tool it is often seen as, but rather is in many respects a tao, or way of thinking, about the world in order to deal with uncertainty (or in other words, life!). Once you understand the Tao of Boyd, you'll find yourself using it more and more in your daily life.

Observe

"If we don't communicate with the outside world – to gain information for knowledge and understanding – we die out to become a non-discerning and uninteresting part of that world." – *John Boyd*

The first step in the OODA Loop is to observe. This is the step that allows us to overcome the 2nd Law of Thermodynamics.

By observing and taking into account new information about our changing environment, our minds become an open system rather than a closed one, and we are able to gain the knowledge and understanding that's crucial in forming new mental models. As an open system, we're positioned to overcome confusion-inducing mental entropy.

From a tactical standpoint, to effectively observe you need to have good situational awareness. You need to always be in Condition Yellow. Condition Yellow is best described as relaxed alert. There's no specific threat situation, but you have your head up and eyes open, and you're taking in your surroundings in a relaxed, but alert manner. I plan on doing a post later this year on improving your situational awareness, but here are a couple things you can start doing now to improve your "A-Game."

Start keying in on where all the exits are whenever you enter a public building. If, heaven forbid, a person enters with guns blazing, you want to know where their possible entry and exit points are and you want to know where your closest exits are located.

Give the people around you the once over and be on the lookout for behavior that doesn't seem "normal." Normal will depend on the situation and environment (having adequate mental models will be important in determining baseline behavior — see "Orient" below), so just because someone is acting weird doesn't necessarily mean they're a threat. Just keep them on your radar.

From a big picture strategic level, say, running a successful business, observation will require you to keep track of not just your gross revenue, expenses, and profit, but also larger trends that may or may not affect your bottom line.

Reading trade journals or blogs related to your business should be part of your regular observations, as well as simply talking to other business owners in not only your own industry but also those that affect yours.

For example, while I should obviously have a depth of knowledge about blogging, I also need to know about web hosting, net neutrality, and other more technical issues that ultimately affect how AoM runs and operates.

In his presentations, Boyd notes that we'll encounter two problems in the Observation phase:

We often observe imperfect or incomplete information (thanks to Heisenberg's Uncertainty Principle);

We can be inundated with so much information that separating the signal from the noise becomes difficult.

These two pitfalls are solved by developing our judgment – our practical wisdom.

As John Boyd scholar Frans P.B. Osinga notes in "Science, Strategy, and War,"

"even if one has perfect information it is of no value if it is not coupled to a penetrating understanding of its meaning, if one does not see the patterns. Judgment is key. Without judgment, data means nothing. It is not necessarily the one with more information who will come out victorious, it is the one with better judgment, the one who is better at discerning patterns."

How do we develop this judgment so that we can better understand our observations? By becoming deft practitioners of the next step in the OODA Loop: Orient.

Orient

The most important step in the OODA Loop, but one that often gets overlooked, is Orient. Boyd called this step the schwerpunkt (a word he borrowed from the German Blitzkrieg), or focal point of the loop.

The reason Orient is the schwerpunkt of the OODA Loop is because that's where our mental models exist, and it is our mental models that shape how everything in the OODA Loop works. As Osinga notes, "orientation shapes the way we interact with the environment…it shapes the way we observe, the way we decide, the way we act. In this sense, orientation shapes the character of present OODA loops, while the present loop shapes the character of future orientation."

So how does one orient himself in a rapidly changing environment?

You constantly have to break apart your old paradigms and put the resulting pieces back together to create a new perspective that better matches your current reality.

Boyd calls this process "destructive deduction." When we do this, we analyze and pull apart our mental concepts into discrete parts. Once we have these constitutive elements, we can start the process of "creative induction" – using these old fragments to form new mental concepts that more closely align with what we have observed is really happening around us.

To illustrate this process, Boyd offered this thought experiment in a presentation called **Strategic Game of ? and ?** (he actually had question marks in his working notes of this presentation and he never filled them in during his career):

"Imagine that you are on a ski slope with other skiers… that you are in Florida riding in an outboard motorboat, maybe even towing water-skiers. Imagine that you are riding a bicycle on a nice spring day.

Imagine that you are a parent taking your son to a department store and that you notice he is fascinated by the toy tractors or tanks with rubber caterpillar treads.

Now imagine that you pull the skis off but you are still on the ski slope. Imagine also that you remove the outboard motor from the motorboat, and you are no longer in Florida. And from the bicycle you remove the handle-bar and discard the rest of the bike.

Finally, you take off the rubber treads from the toy tractor or tanks. This leaves only the following separate pieces: skis, outboard motor, handlebars and rubber treads."

Boyd then challenged his audience to imagine what emerges when you put these particular parts together.

Did you figure it out?

It's a snowmobile.

Orienting, in a nutshell, is the ability to make figurative mental snowmobiles on the fly and in the face of uncertainty.

According to Boyd, the ability to orient effectively is what separated the winners from the losers in any conflict:

"A loser is someone (individual or group) who cannot build snowmobiles when facing uncertainty and unpredictable change; whereas a winner is someone (individual or group) who can build snowmobiles, and employ them in an appropriate fashion, when facing uncertainty and unpredictable change."

It's important to point out that deductive destruction and creative induction of mental models isn't a one-time event. For Boyd, it's a continual process; as soon as you create that new mental concept, it will quickly become outdated as the environment around you changes.

So if Orientation is the key to successfully implementing the OODA Loop, how can we become better at it?

Boyd left us with some ideas:

1. Build a robust toolbox of mental models.

The more mental models you have at your disposal, the more you have to work with in creating new ones.

During a presentation at the Air War College in 1992, Boyd warned his audience of the way in which strict operational doctrines can stifle the cultivation of a robust toolbox of mental models:

"The Air Force has got a doctrine, the Army's got a doctrine, Navy's got a doctrine, everybody's got a doctrine. [But if you] read my work, 'doctrine' doesn't appear in there even once. You can't find it. You know why I don't have it in there? Because it's doctrine on day one, and every day after it becomes dogma. That's why…."

Doctrines have the tendency to harden into dogmas, and dogmatism has the tendency to create folks with "man with a hammer syndrome" – it causes people to keep trying to apply that same old mental model even if it's no longer applicable to the changing environment. You see "man with a hammer syndrome" in businesses that stick to a tried and tested business model even though the market is moving in another direction.

Kodak, as mentioned above, is a perfect example of this. So too is Blockbuster. They continued making hard-copy movie rental a primary part of their business even though more and more consumers were streaming movies via the internet. Blockbuster eventually tried to shift their business model, but it was too little, too late.

You also see "man with a hammer syndrome" in folks who discover some pet theory and start applying it to every single situation in life without considering other factors.

People who are fans of evolutionary psychology are prone to this. To them, all human behavior can be explained by it. Why are men more jealous than women? Because in primitive times they couldn't know if they were really the father of a baby or not. Why do we get depressed? It used to help people concentrate on their problems and figure out how to remove themselves from a bad situation. While our evolved psychology certainly plays a big role in our behavior, other factors are also involved in why we do what we do. It's foolish to discount those.

It's for this reason that Boyd advocated for familiarizing yourself with as many theories and fields of knowledge as possible, and continuing to challenge your beliefs, even when you think you've got them figured out:

"Well, I understand you're going to have to write [military] doctrine, and that's all right… [But] even after you write it, assume it's not right. And look at a whole lot of other doctrines – German doctrine, other kinds of doctrines – and learn those too. And then you've got a bunch of doctrines, and the reason you want to learn them all [is so that] you're not captured by any one, and you can lift stuff out of here, stuff out of there…. You can put your snowmobile [together], and you do better than anyone else. If you got one doctrine, you're a dinosaur. Period."

The more doctrines, or mental models, we have at our mental fingertips, the more materials we have from which to construct our figurative snowmobiles.

Charlie Munger advanced a similar argument for the necessity of having a widely varied library of mental knowledge in a speech he gave at the USC Business School in 1994:

"You've got to have models in your head. And you've got to array your experience — both vicarious and direct — on this lattice work of models. You may have noticed students who just try to remember and pound back what is remembered. Well, they fail in school and in life. You've got to hang experience on a lattice work of models in your head. What are the models? Well, the first rule is that you've got to have multiple models — because if you just have one or two that you're using, the nature of human psychology is such that you'll torture reality so that it fits your models, or at least you'll think it does…So you've got to have multiple models. And the models have to come from multiple disciplines — because all the wisdom of the world is not to be found in one little academic department."

Munger has repeatedly emphasized in his speeches that reality is an interconnected ecosystem of factors that influence one another. Thus, to understand this ecosystem, you need to apply multiple models in an interconnected fashion. John Muir put it best when he noted: "When we try to pick out anything by itself, we find it hitched to everything else in the universe."

So all this talk of having multiple mental models begs the question: what sort of models should you put in your toolbox?

Both Boyd and Munger give some suggestions. In his presentation of **Strategic Game of ? and ?**, Boyd lays out seven disciplines every military strategist (or any person strategizing how to win any kind of conflict or competition) ought to know:

>Mathematical Logic
>Physics
>Thermodynamics
>Biology
>Psychology
>Anthropology
>Conflict (Game Theory)

Boyd emphasized that his list was of course not exhaustive and that other mental concepts should be pursued as well. In other presentations, Boyd hinted that biological evolution and quantum mechanics are additional mental models every master strategist should have a grasp of.

Munger's list includes the following mental models:

Math
(Munger is particularly fond of the algebraic idea of inversion, that is, to solve a problem you address it backwards)

Accounting
(and its limits)

Engineering
(according to Munger, the ideas of redundancies and break-points are applicable outside of engineering and can be applied to business)

Economics

Probability

Psychology
(specifically the cognitive biases that cause us to make terrible decisions)

Chemistry

Evolutionary biology
(can provide insights into economics)

History

Statistics

I would personally add philosophy, literature (and its accompanying models of interpretation), and basic common law principles (like torts, contract law, and property law) to the list.

Because Boyd and Munger are thinking "Big Picture," their mental model examples are purposely general and abstract. But it's important to remember that mental models can be specific and concrete.

To thrive in your job, you'll need certain mental models specific to your career. To survive a lethal encounter, you'll need certain mental models unique to tactical situations. Learn as many mental models as you can, and create as exhaustive a lattice work as possible, so you have more to work with in the creation and destruction process.

Some of these subjects can certainly be intimidating for people with no experience in them. To get started, take a look at the resources section in our article on lifelong learning – particularly the online courses. Coursera, for instance, has a number of introductory classes on calculus, econ, competitive strategy, etc.

2. Start destroying and creating mental models.

Your fluency in destroying and creating mental models will only come with practice, so start doing it as much as you can. When you're faced with a new problem, go through the domains above in a checklist-like fashion and ask yourself, "Are there elements from these different mental concepts that can provide insight into my problem?"

Perhaps there's a principle from engineering, the works of Plato, and biology that can help create a new mental model that matches up with your new reality.
Start a journal with your destruction and creation experiments. Suss out new mental concepts with writing and doodles. You may be surprised by the insights you'll gain from this exercise.

As you practice destroying and creating mental models, you'll find that it will become easier and easier to do on the fly. It will become almost intuitive. In Mastery, Robert Greene described the great military strategists from history as having a "fingertip feel" for knowing how to proceed on the battlefield. These great strategists simply were effective and efficient at orienting. They didn't have to deliberately think about the process, they just did it. That should be your goal.

3. Never stop orienting.

"Orientation isn't just a state you're in; it's a process. You're always orienting." — *John Boyd*

Because the world around you is constantly changing, orientation is something you can never stop doing. "ABO = Always Be Orienting" should become your mantra. Make it a goal to add to your toolbox of mental models every day, and then immediately start atomizing those models and fashioning new ones.

4. Try to validate mental models before operation.

Ideally, according to Boyd, you want to be fairly confident that your mental models or concepts will work before you actually need to use them. This is especially true in combat or life-or-death situations where rapid cycling of the OODA Loop is crucial.

How do you validate mental models before operation? You study what mental concepts have and haven't worked in similar situations and then practice, train, and visualize using those mental concepts. Think of the situation where a basketball team is losing the game by one basket, there's just seconds left on the clock, and they're inbounding the ball. They've already spent weeks practicing specific plays designed for these specific circumstances and now they just have to execute that plan.

Having field-tested mental concepts at the ready is important even when time isn't of the essence. In business, you can read case studies of what has and hasn't worked for other companies and have models, concepts, and strategies at the ready that you can implement immediately when similar situations arise. Of course, if those don't work, you'll need to continue the process of orientation until you create a new mental model better suited for the situation.

When your observations about your environment match up with certain proven mental models, you don't have to do any destroying and creating, you just have to act.

A person who has achieved mastery in a specific domain should be able to quickly notice when reality lines up with a specific mental model and then execute that mental model without having to decide. You just act.

I can't hit home hard enough the importance of the orientation step. It's at the heart of the OODA Loop and is what determines your successful implementation of it. If you don't act with the mental model that matches up closest to your environment, you're going to lose no matter how quickly you cycle through the Loop. ABO = Always Be Orienting.

Decide

Boyd doesn't articulate much about the decision step except that it's the "component in which actors decide among action alternatives generated in the Orientation phase."

For Boyd, it's impossible to select a perfectly matching mental model because:

1. We often have imperfect information of our environment

2. Even if we had perfect information, Heisenberg's Uncertainty Principle prevents us from attaining a perfect match-up between our environment and our mental model.

Consequently, when we decide which mental model(s) to use, we're forced to settle for ones that aren't perfect, but good enough.

It's interesting to note that in his final sketch of the OODA Loop, Boyd put "Hypothesis" in parentheses next to "Decide," suggesting the uncertain nature of our decisions. When we decide, we're essentially moving forward with our best hypothesis — our best "educated guess" — about which mental model will work. To find out if our hypothesis is correct, we then have to test it, which takes us to our next step:

Act
Once you've decided on a mental concept to implement, you must act.

In his final sketch of the OODA Loop, Boyd has "Test" next to "Act," again indicating that the OODA Loop is not only a decision process, but a learning system; we are all like scientists perpetually testing our new hypotheses in the real world. We should all be constantly "experimenting," and gaining new "data" that improves how we operate in every facet of our lives. As Osinga notes in "Science, Strategy, and War," actions "feed back into the systems as validity checks on the correctness and adequacy of the existing orientation patterns."

Action is how we find out if our mental models are correct. If they are, we win the battle; if they aren't, then we start the OODA Loop again using our newly observed data.

Ideally, you'll have multiple actions/tests/experiments going on at the same time so that you can quickly discover the best mental model for a particular situation. In war, this might mean having multiple attack points that are using different weapons systems. When the strategist discovers which targets and weapons are providing the best results, he'll direct his attention to the winning mental model and exploit it to the max until it no longer works.

Once he observes that it is no longer effective, he'll orient more mental concepts, decide to use one or several of them, and quickly act to test them out. Over and over this process goes until the enemy is eliminated.

The same goes in business. Ideally, you'll want to try out different strategies at the same time to see which ones work. A/B testing is a good example of this. In A/B testing, marketers or online publications will come up with multiple headlines or copy (orientation!) and deploy them on different segments of their audience at the same time.

They'll then sit back and watch which headline, message, etc. performs the best. Whichever headline gets the most clicks will then become the default.

"We gotta get an image or picture in our head, which we call orientation. Then we have to make a decision as to what we're going to do, and then implement the decision….Then we look at the [resulting] action, plus our observation, and we drag in new data, new orientation, new decision, new action, ad infinitum…"
— *John Boyd "Tempo: To the Swift Goes the Race"*

"Under OODA loop theory every combatant observes the situation, orients himself…decides what to do and then does it. If his opponent can do this faster, however, his own actions become outdated and disconnected to the true situation, and his opponent's advantage increases geometrically." — John Boyd

Throughout this chapter, we've been talking about the OODA Loop largely as a learning system that can be employed in any uncertain situation in order to figure out the best course of action to take and how to proceed. It can guide our individual actions and doesn't require an "opponent" per se in order to be useful.

But the tool can also be used in situations of conflict and competition, where it's your OODA Loop going head-to-head against someone else's. Indeed, this is what the OODA Loop is most famously employed for. Each individual or group is trying to work its way through the Loop more quickly and effectively than their competitors.

For this reason, understanding the basic principles for how the OODA Loop works isn't enough to successfully implement it. Tempo is also a vital underlying element.

When I met with Curtis Sprague, former US Air Marshal and instructor, he told me that there are two general principles to keep in mind when considering tempo and the OODA Loop.

First, the individual or organization that can go through successful, consecutive OODA Loops faster than their opponent will win the conflict.

Second, rapid OODA Looping on your part "resets" your opponent's OODA Loop by causing confusion — it sends them back to square one; back to the observation phase; back to figuring out how to proceed. This delay provides you more time to complete your OODA Loop before your opponent does.

For example, when Boise State busted out three trick plays — the hook-and-lateral, the Statue of Liberty, and the halfback toss – during the 2007 Fiesta Bowl, it reset the University of Oklahoma's OODA Loop (along with that of the entirety of the Sooner Nation); OU was caught flat-footed and couldn't re-orient quickly enough to surmount the Broncos surge.

To show the vital importance of controlling the tempo of your OODA Loop when it clashes with another's, Curtis pointed to the door of the coffee shop at which we were meeting, and asked me, "What would you do if a guy with a gun came in through that door?"

Me: "Uhhh…."

"You're dead. You got stuck in the orientation step. You need to have a plan that you know is good enough to work in that situation and implement it immediately. Remember, you have to finish your Loop before the bad guy finishes his."

So what's the best mental model in that situation? According to Curtis, as well as research on past active shootings (or active murders, as Lt. Col. Grossman calls them), the best response isn't to flee or hide from the gunman, but rather to immediately close the gap between you and him and incapacitate him. In fact, this is what Homeland Security recommends when the shooter is relatively close to you.

Why does this work? When you immediately go after the shooter, you're messing up his plan and his orientation of the world. You're getting inside his OODA Loop, or as Curtis says, you're "resetting it":

"Most violent gunmen think that because they have the gun, people will do what they say and will just hide. They don't expect someone to come charging after them. By closing the gap, you're resetting your adversary's Loop because now they have to re-orient themselves to an unexpected change in the environment. You're making them have an 'uhhhh…' moment. By causing the reset, you've slowed him down, even if it's just by a few seconds, which gives you more time to complete your OODA Loop and win the battle."

In order for you to implement a mental model with this kind of rapidity, you have to practice it. "The body can't go where the brain hasn't been," said Curtis. "You need to practice and visualize yourself closing the gap in an active shooter situation before it actually happens if you want to be able to implement it in real life. If you don't, you'll just end up freezing."

So fast cycling of your OODA Loop can allow you to get inside, or reset, your opponent's, which allows you to complete your Loop first and win the fight. Speed is relative in the OODA Loop. You just have to be faster than the person you're competing against.

But simply cycling through your OODA Loop as fast as you can is an incomplete picture of tempo. What often gets overlooked by folks studying the OODA Loop is that when Boyd talked about rapid tempo, he often meant rapid changes in tempo.

He argued that when it comes to winning a competition or conflict, our actions need to be surprising, ambiguous, and varying; speeding up and slowing down your actions quickly and irregularly can create confusion just as much and sometimes more than simply blowing through your OODA Loop. If the enemy is expecting a sudden and quick attack from you, but you instead delay, you may cause your enemy to have an "uhhh..." moment that can be exploited.

What's more, when you move from a boots-on-the-ground tactical level to a bigger picture strategic level, Boyd puts less emphasis on fast OODA Looping and instead focuses on developing the best mental concepts possible to win the battle or war.

It's at this "big picture" level, when a strategist is playing the long-game, that he takes into account domains like politics, culture, economics, diplomacy, and espionage. In this long game, his time interval to complete the OODA Loop becomes longer.

He still has to complete his strategic Loop before the enemy's or competitor's, but he has a longer timeframe to do it compared to the foot soldier that's actually engaged in the heat of battle.

Conclusion

The OODA Loop makes explicit our implicit decision-making process. By making it explicit, Boyd offered an incomparable strategic tool to everyone from soldiers and militaries to businesses and sports teams to social movement leaders and political campaigners to better manage their own decision-making processes.

It also allows the manipulation and control of the decision-making process of our competitors. Controlling both your own and your enemy's OODA Loops allows you to come off conqueror. In addition to being a tool to vanquish your foe, the OODA Loop is a learning engine that allows an individual or organization to thrive in a changing environment.

Ever since I started researching the OODA Loop, I've gained new insights in a whole host of areas. By knowing that the key to success in a violent confrontation is getting through your OODA Loop faster and resetting the bad guy's Loop, whenever I'm out, I'm always "orienting" by thinking about what I would do if some bad dude suddenly appeared. I've taken to following General James Mattis's advice to Marines: "Be polite, be professional, but have a plan to kill everybody you meet."

Understanding the OODA Loop has also helped me become more strategic about my business. Online publishing is a relatively new industry and the technology that supports it is always changing.

I've even been able to apply the OODA Loop to better understand current affairs.

Take what's going in Ukraine or in the Middle East with ISIS. The actions by Putin (invading a sovereign country) and ISIS (beheading journalists, etc.) have caused the U.S. and other Western countries to have an "uhhhh.." moment. Putin and ISIS have effectively reset America's OODA Loop through quick and unexpected actions. Putin effectively employs unpredictable tempo – making quick moves, or saying bold things, and then appearing to draw back.

Western politicians and militaries are having to come up with new mental models or strategies for how to react to a powerful country invading another, as well as needing to figure out how to respond to an amorphous terrorist organization that wants to fly their flag from the top of the White House.

As some Joe Schmo, I have no influence on how things turn out in those political and military arenas, but it's interesting nonetheless to see the OODA Loop play out on the world stage.

Don't be fooled by the simplicity of the OODA Loop – it has the power and potential to change your life. As you start looking at your life through the lens of the Loop, you'll gain insights about how to achieve success that you otherwise would be oblivious to.

Follow the Tao of Boyd, and you'll be able to do something in this life and not just be somebody.

Sources:

Science, Strategy, and War by Frans P.B. Osinga (The best resource on John Boyd's work. It's expensive, but if you really want to dig into the development of the OODA Loop, it's a must read.

The Mind of War: John Boyd and American Security by Grant Hammond

Boyd: The Fighter Pilot Who Changed the Art of War by Robert Coram

A Vision So Noble by Daniel Ford

Curtis Sprague of Dark Horse Tactical. His insights on how to apply the Loop in tactical situations was invaluable.

CHAPTER EIGHT

What to do in an Active Shooter Situation

(Editor's note) This chapter is the essay, "What to do in an active shooter situation," written by Brett and Kate McKay, and published on the website artofmanliness.com. It is used with permission of the authors, and includes important pointers on surviving an active shooter situation.

It's a sad fact of life in the 21st century that active shootings have become a regular occurrence in the United States. In other parts of the world, terrorist groups are using active shootings to, well, terrorize.

While the media focuses on the firestorm of political debate these events cyclically create, I've rarely seen them discuss what people are actually supposed to do in these situations.

According to the FBI, active shootings in public places are becoming increasingly common. Which means it would serve everyone to understand how to respond if they ever find themselves in the line of fire.

Over the years I've talked to a lot of military, tactical, and law enforcement professionals who've spent their careers training and dealing with violent individuals: U.S. marshals, SWAT officers, and special forces operators. And I've asked them all this same question: What's an average joe civilian like me supposed to do when faced with a gunman who's indiscriminately firing on people?

They've all answered the same way.

In this article, I share expert-backed advice on how best to react if you ever find yourself in a situation with an active shooter. Learning how to survive a shooting is much like learning how to survive an airplane crash: such an event is statistically unlikely to happen to you, and simple chance may make you a victim before you're able to take any volitional action. But if there are things you can do to increase your odds of survival even slightly, you ought to know and practice them.

Something to Keep in Mind: You're Probably On Your Own!

In a study done by the FBI in 2014, it was discovered that most active shootings end in 2 minutes or less. That's not enough time for law enforcement to arrive. So when you start hearing gunshots in places you shouldn't be hearing gunshots, understand that you don't have very much time to think about what you should do.

That's why... You've Got to Know What You'd Do Before It Actually Happens.

When any sort of emergency situation strikes, be it an active shooter or even a fire, the natural response for most people, surprisingly enough, is not to do anything. Most people freeze up in emergency situations. For example, the "normalcy bias" causes victims to act like everything is fine even though things are far from it.

Our brain is predisposed to assume that things will carry on in a predictable way. When the pattern is broken, it takes a long time for the brain to process this aberration. This is why many people who witness traumatic events report that it felt surreal, like they were watching a movie and it wasn't really happening. They also often say that at first they thought the gunshots were fireworks or a car backfiring or a book falling — things that would fit better in their usual paradigm of daily life.

Another bias that keeps us from taking action is our natural tendency to follow the crowd. If we see that everyone else is cowering in fear or locked up by inertia, then our natural tendency is to act the same.

The way you overcome these inclinations towards passivity is deciding exactly what you'll do in the event of a shooting — before one ever happens. You've got to have a plan.

I know it seems morbid, but you really should visualize what you would do in various situations were an active shooter to suddenly intrude upon the scene.

What would your plan be if you were in the office and heard shots coming from the floor beneath you? Would you have time to run? If so, where would you go? If you heard the shots just down the hallway and there's no place to run or hide, what would be your next step? Visualize your plan in as much detail as possible.

In an active shooter situation, seconds matter. You don't have time to figure out what you're going to do when a guy starts spraying a building full of gunfire. By having a general preconceived plan, you give yourself a head start. This all goes back to the chapter on the OODA Loop. Remember, in any conflict there are multiple loops going on. It's your loop versus the shooter's, and the first to complete their respective decision-making cycle usually wins the fight.

OODA Loops can begin way before an actual encounter starts. By coming up with a plan of what you would do in an active shooter situation before one ever happens, you're already engaged in the second step: Orienting. Should you encounter a shooter, you can act immediately because you've already begun the cycle and already have a plan in place. Remember, ABO = Always Be Orienting.

Maintain Situational Awareness Wherever You Go

Besides having a general idea of what you'd do in an active shooter situation, another thing you must do to increase your chances of surviving is constantly maintaining situational awareness.

We've written in detail about situational awareness before, so rather than getting into the nitty gritty here, let's review a few important principles as they apply to shootings:

Stay in Condition Yellow. Condition Yellow is best described as "relaxed alert."

There's no specific threat situation, but you have your head up and you're taking in your surroundings with all your senses. Most people associate situational awareness with just visual stimulation, but you can also learn a lot about a particular scenario from sounds.

This is especially true for active shootings. If you hear gunshots — or something that sounds an awful lot like gunshots — that should be a sign that you need to start immediately preparing to take action.

Though your senses are slightly heightened in Condition Yellow, it's also important to stay relaxed. Staying relaxed ensures that you maintain an open focus, which allows you to take in more information about what's going on around you.

Research shows that when we get nervous or stressed, our attention narrows, causing us to concentrate on just a few things at a time. A narrow focus can therefore cause us to miss important details in our environment.

Bottom line: Don't have your nose constantly in your smartphone and don't zone out; rather, you should open your eyes, ears, and nose, and calmly and constantly scan your environment to take in what's going on.

Establish baselines and look for anomalies. As Patrick Van Horne notes in his book "Left of Bang," a key component of situational awareness is establishing baselines and looking for anomalies.

A baseline is what's "normal" in a given situation, and it will differ from person to person and environment to environment. A baseline in an office would be people working at their desks or chatting in a lobby. A baseline at a restaurant would be people in uniforms coming in and out of the kitchen and customers entering and exiting the restaurant through the front door.

We establish baselines so that we can look for anomalies. Hearing gunshots at a college campus is definitely out of the ordinary, and should immediately trigger your active shooter plan of action. But let's take a look at a subtler anomaly.

If you're at a movie theater and you see a guy entering the theater from the exit near the screen, that should definitely put you on alert. It could just be a guy sneaking in for a free movie, but it could also be a gunman. You don't need to go and immediately tackle the guy, but you'd certainly want to keep your eye on him and make sure you're prepared to quickly move out.

Know where all your exits are. If there's one actionable takeaway you get from this article, let it be this. *Wherever you are, always know the locations of the nearest exits.*

As we'll see in a moment, running should be your first line of action in an active shooter situation. You want to get as far away from the gunman as possible and that often means getting out of the building where he's shooting. So whenever you enter a building, the first thing you should do is look for exit signs and make mental notes of them.

You also need to consider not-so-visible exits. For example, most grocery stores will have an exit door in the very back in the "employee only" section. If you're near the back of the store and you hear gunshots from the front, you'll want to head directly to this rear exit.

Another example of not-so-obvious exits is in restaurants. Most restaurants will have an exit in the back of the kitchen. If you're near the kitchen and you hear gunshots near the front of the place, you'd want to hightail it to this back door. Because these exits are in places considered "employee only," people have been conditioned not to even consider using them. But in an active shooter situation, these kinds of norms obviously go out the window, and preparing yourself to disregard them is a must.

Your Active Shooter Triage: Run, Hide, Fight

So you've heard shots and screams. There's an active shooting happening. What should you do? All the experts agree that you have three possible actions: run, hide, and fight.

Run

Running away should always be your first line of action. As soon as you hear gunfire, leave the premises immediately using your preconceived escape plan and get as far away from the shooter as possible. Ideally, you'll be able to escape without having to cross the shooter's path.

Keep in mind that in an active shooter situation, most people won't want to leave because 1) they're cowed in fear, 2) they've let the normalcy bias take over, or 3) they think hiding should be their first recourse. But you need to run, regardless of what others are doing. Do all you can to convince them to come with you, but if they don't comply, leave them, and get out of the building or danger area as soon as possible.

Don't try to gather your belongings. You can replace your laptop; you can't replace your life.

As you make your exit, tell others to come along with you. Once you're out of the danger area, prevent others (except for law enforcement) from entering the premises.

When you're running, keep your hands visible. Law enforcement will be checking you to decide if you're a threat.

This may go against every humane compulsion you have, but don't try to move or assist the wounded while you're making your exit. It leaves you vulnerable to attack; turning one casualty into two won't ultimately help things.

Even the first law enforcement officers to arrive at the scene will initially ignore the wounded so they can take out the shooter. Just as their top priority is to stop the gunman, your top priority is to get to safety.

If you're in an open area and there's distance between you and the shooter, run as fast as you can in a zig-zag pattern. Shooting a moving target is hard even for experienced marksman, and many mass shooters have little or no experience with firearms. So move as much as possible and take cover behind barriers that can stop bullets (cement pillars, vending machines, etc.).

As soon as you get to safety, call 911. Don't assume someone already has.

Hide

Sometimes running isn't an option. Maybe the shooter is in front of the only exit and you can't jump out the window because you're on the fourth floor. If you can't make an escape, the next best thing to do is to hide in a secure location.

You want to hide in a place that's out of the shooter's view and that can provide protection if shots are fired in your direction.

If you're in an office or school building, find a room that has a lockable door. If you can't lock the door of the room you're in, barricade it with a table and chairs. You want to make it as hard as possible for the shooter to enter; he's often looking for easy victims, and will move on rather than bother pushing through the barrier.

Turn off the lights in the room and be as quiet as possible. Be sure to put your cell phone on silent. You don't even want it on vibrate.

Stay away from the door and crouch behind items that could offer protection from bullets like cabinets or desks. Hide in a bathroom or closet if you can.

If possible, dial 911 and let the authorities know there's an active shooter in your building. If you can't speak because the shooter is nearby, leave the line open so the dispatcher can hear what's going on.

Don't open the door unless absolutely necessary or if you can confirm it's the authorities who are knocking.

According to Clint Emerson, Navy SEAL and author of the book "100 Deadly Skills," shooters will often knock on doors or yell for help in the hopes of convincing people who are hiding to show themselves.

If you can't find a room in which to secure yourself, hide in a location that offers cover and concealment from the shooter, but still allows you to see him. If the shooter passes you, you can make a run for it. If he doesn't, it puts you in a position to attack if necessary.

Fight!

When running or hiding have failed or aren't viable options, it's time to resort to plan C: which is to Fight!

Most civilians don't think they can take on an active shooter because, well, the shooter has a gun and they likely do not. But here's the thing: It is possible for unarmed individuals to subdue or chase away an armed shooter.

Anthony Sadler, Spencer Stone, and Alek Skarlatos —
the three friends who rushed a terrorist aboard a train to
Paris — did it, saving dozens of lives.

So did Frank Hall, a football coach who ran down a
shooter and chased him out of a high school in Ohio
before he could wreak massive carnage.

Yes, some studies have suggested that armed civilians
can reduce the number of fatalities in an active shooter
situation compared to situations where there were no
armed civilians.

But what these same studies suggest is that just having
civilians — armed or not — quickly take action against
a shooter can reduce the number of victims too. So even
if you don't plan on carrying a firearm yourself, commit
to the idea that if you absolutely have to (and, again,
we're talking last resort here), you'll attack an active
shooter quickly and devastatingly.

Will you get shot? Possibly. But it's possible to survive
multiple gunshot wounds, and doing nothing will
probably get you killed anyway. Sadly, history has
shown that many active shooters will unflinchingly
shoot people begging for their lives while they're curled
up in the fetal position. As Chris Norman, a Briton who
assisted the three Americans in their attack of the train
terrorist described his reason for taking action:

"My thought was, 'OK, I'm probably going to die
anyway, so let's go.' I'd rather die being active, trying to
get him down, than simply sit in the corner and be shot.

Either you sit down and you die or you get up and you die. It was really nothing more than that."

How to Fight an Active Shooter

So you've made the decision that running and hiding are no longer options and that fighting is your last recourse. What's the best way to fight an active shooter?

If you're armed yourself, there are certain techniques you should employ in returning fire. A tutorial on how to take down a gunman lies outside the purview of this chapter, and must be practiced in the real world.

If you're not armed, real world practice in hand-to-hand fighting will be an enormous asset, not only in giving you concrete skills to employ, but in offering you a greater comfort level with violence and a confidence in taking action.

It's not a coincidence that Spencer Stone — a U.S. Airman who was the first of the three Americans to rush the train-bound terrorist and choked him out while his buddies gave him a beat down — was trained in Brazilian Jiu-Jitsu.

Stone unequivocally attributed his training in martial arts to his survival, adding that even a cursory knowledge of self-defense is highly beneficial:

"I 100% believe that Brazilian Jiu-Jitsu saved my life at that moment. Every move I used on him was very, very basic — you can learn in five minutes. If we had a course like that in the Air Force for people to learn basic moves, it could help anyone in a situation like that."

But even if you're the most average of average Joes — you've got neither a gun nor a black belt — you should still attempt to take on a gunman as a last resort, keeping these principles in mind:

Understand your advantages. Most violent gunmen work under the assumption that because they have a gun, people will do what they want or just hide. They don't expect someone to come charging after them.

As we discussed in our article on the OODA Loop, an important part of winning any fight is resetting or disrupting your opponent's loop. As former US Air Marshal Curtis Sprague told me, you want your opponent to have an "uhhhh…" moment. By doing the unexpected (attacking), Sprague argues that "you're disrupting the gunman's OODA Loop which slows him down — even if it's just a few seconds — and gives you more time to complete your OODA Loop and win the battle."

So simply charging your gunman puts you at an advantage because he's definitely not expecting it.

In "100 Deadly Skills," Emerson notes another advantage to keep in mind: "a gun can only be shot in one direction at any one time." If you approach the shooter from behind or from the side, it's going to be very hard for him to shoot you. What's more, if you attack the shooter as a team (which you should), he can't shoot everyone at the same time. An attack by multiple people, from multiple angles, will be difficult for a lone gunman to fend off.

Be aggressive and violent. This isn't the time for pussy footing. Once you decide to fight, attack with violence and aggression.

Alek Skarlatos grabbed the train-bound terrorist's rifle and pounded him repeatedly in the head with its muzzle. This kind of violence may not be pleasant to contemplate, but remember, old ingrained norms like never hurting others go out the window in a crisis; victory will go to the swift and relentless. Use lethal force, and don't stop fighting until you're dead or the shooter stops moving.

Control the weapon and then control the shooter. The sooner you can get the weapon out of the shooter's hands, without endangering others, the better. Without his gun, he can't shoot anymore. Once the weapon has been secured, turn your attention to completely containing the perpetrator.

Keep in mind every fight is different. Sometimes you're not going to be in a position to secure the weapon first, so your priority would be to inflict as much violence as possible on the shooter until you can get the gun away from him.

Even if you can't get the gun completely out of the attacker's hands, do what you can to control it. Grab the gun so that you can exercise some influence over where it's pointed. If the shooter has a semi-automatic pistol, use this tip I picked up from UFC fighter and Army

Ranger Tim Kennedy at the Atomic Athlete Vanguard. Grab the barrel as hard as you can. First, this allows you to control where the gun is pointed. And second, if the gun does fire, it will prevent the slide from going back and chambering another round, thus preventing the shooter from re-firing.

Use improvised weapons. Just because you don't have a gun, doesn't mean you don't have a weapon. A weapon can multiply force and almost anything in your environment can be turned into one: Chairs, fire extinguishers, umbrellas, belts, coffee mugs. Heck, even a pen can be used as an improvised weapon.

Throw stuff at the shooter. Even if it doesn't disable him, you're creating hesitation which will give you more time to get closer to end the fight. Remember, disrupt that loop!

If it's available, use items that can blind the shooter: flash a high-beam tactical flashlight in his eyes, spray a fire extinguisher or chemicals in his face, or throw a pot of scalding hot coffee his way. Be creative! Once the shooter is disoriented, rush him and take him down.

Work as a team. The more people you can get to help you in attacking the shooter, the better your chances of ending the ordeal with fewer casualties.

But remember, most people's natural reaction in these sorts of situations is to not do anything. You'll need to be assertive and take the lead. Courage is contagious.

Conclusion

While active shootings are increasing, they're still rare. We shouldn't be cowered in our homes in fear. But there's no downside to being prepared.

Sometimes there's nothing you can do to survive a shooting; you're in the wrong place, at the wrong time, and you're killed without warning. But you may get a chance to act, and will only have seconds to figure out what to do.

Your stress will be through the roof and the situation will be utter chaos. If you hope in that moment to be able to protect your life and the lives of others, ready yourself now and have a plan of action wherever you go.

Sources:
100 Deadly Skills by Clint Emerson
Left of Bang by Patrick van Horne
How to Survive the Most Critical 5 Seconds of Your Life by Tim Larkin
Active Shooter: How to Respond by The Department of Homeland Security

CHAPTER NINE

Personal security and the Internet

Doxing (from dox, abbreviation of documents) or doxxing is the Internet-based practice of researching and broadcasting private or identifiable information (especially personally identifiable information) about an individual or organization.

The methods employed to acquire this information include searching publicly available databases and social media websites (like Facebook), hacking, and social engineering. It is closely related to Internet vigilantism and hacktivism.

Doxing may be carried out for various reasons, including to aid law enforcement, business analysis, risk analytics, extortion, coercion, inflict harm, harassment, online shaming, and vigilante justice.

Eva Galperin, on wired.com, says "Generally people don't think about this stuff until it's too late, so it's good for everyone to have some sort of privacy and security posture set up before things go wrong. Especially if you are about to do something that's going to attract you some attention, but even if you are just a woman on the internet."

For journalists and media people, keeping your personal information separate from your professional online profiles can be difficult, especially using social media platforms such as Facebook or Twitter. But keeping your personal information and life protected from the online public can be crucial.

I have had the experience a few times where a news event I covered became a nation-wide crap magnet, drawing threats and hate mail from all over the country — and my experiences were minor compared to what major celebrities or media personalities might endure.

Doxxing can happen to anyone, and it makes you vulnerable to personal attacks. Even worse, it opens up your family to possible harm.

Galperin continues: "What I tell people is: Google yourself, lock yourself down, make it harder to access information about you.

"People should definitely be aware of their public records, like their public tax records. And when you post your photos to Instagram, or you make posts to Facebook, or you tweet something about your location, people can take that stuff, put it into another context, and suddenly you have been doxed. What people can really give away about you is the stuff that you've already given away about yourself."

Galperin says "think about the possibility in advance, and to have a plan, in the same way that you have a plan for all kinds of other emergencies."

She recommends everyone see what is already available online about you. Be familiar with the Terms of Service of the various platforms you use. Learn how to properly file a takedown for when your information does get up there.

Galperin says "remove your name from people-search lists, take down information about yourself, make sure that your number is unlisted."

Equality Labs has a great, thorough doxing guide that includes a number of opt-out links.

In addition to doxing, everyone should also be concerned about the security of your accounts.

"If you have earned the attention of people who think it is worthwhile to dox you, they may also think it's worthwhile to compromise your security and post things as you, or get more information about you by logging in as you to your accounts, Galperin said.

Definitely have long, strong, unique passwords.

Use a password manager. Use two-factor authentication, and set it up when possible with a security key or an authentication app rather than text messages.

"I would also recommend calling up your cell company and telling them to lock down your account, giving them a password to use so that nobody can hijack your SIM.," she said.

CHAPTER TEN

Cyberbullying and Doxxing

Sameer Hinduja, on the website cyberbullying.org, reports that the Crash Override Network (a task force made up of people who have previously been targeted) describes doxxing as a "tactic of mobs of anonymous online groups" whose goal is to scare targets by exposing their personal information online.

"While your personal information may have nothing to do with them, their objective is to make you fearful about how it could potentially lead to your own victimization," Hinduja writes.

The scariest part, of course, is that once your private contact details are put out there electronically, it's difficult to get them taken down. Therefore the information is available for anyone with malicious or reckless motives to see, find, and use against you.

Doxing first arose in the hacker culture in the 1990s, and recently has been used by journalists to refer to "deep investigative reporting."

A famous case of doxxing involved the killing of Cecil the Lion.

In July of 2015, the Sun Sentinel reported that a lion named Cecil was "lured from a protected national park in Zimbabwe and killed in an illegal hunt." The Telegraph, a prominent British newspaper, then disclosed the identity of the hunter involved — Walter Palmer, a dentist from Minneapolis, Minnesota.

Shortly after Palmer's identity was released, he became the subject of internet hate, being called a "scumbag," "disgrace to humankind" and a "detriment to our species as a whole."

His address, website and work phone number were "plastered everywhere" and his work website was taken offline as a result. Of his own volition, he took his Facebook page down as well. Not only has Palmer had his life threatened online, he has also faced protests outside his office in Minneapolis.

Moreover, his vacation home in Florida was also vandalized, as individuals spray-painted the words "lion killer" on his garage door.

Another case involved Ashley Madison, the online dating site specifically oriented towards those interested in "extramarital romance and sex."

Like Tinder or other online environments in which relationships and hookups are fostered, Ashley Madison users browse through the profiles of others who are seemingly looking to have an affair.

A group of hackers called the "Impact Team" ordered Ashley Madison to permanently take down the site, alleging questionable morals and fraudulent business practices.

When Ashley Madison did not comply, the hacker group released about ten gigabytes of user data from the site. This included around thirty million Ashley Madison user e-mail addresses.

Approximately half of those were military and government addresses.

Users' personal information, such as names, addresses, phone numbers and sexual preferences and interests, were also made public.

Victims of the data leak quickly became concerned about public embarrassment, shame, and their partners finding out. A pastor in New Orleans committed suicide after being outed in this way; he specifically mentioned Ashley Madison in his suicide note.

According to Wikipedia, Cyberstalking is the use of the Internet or other electronic means to stalk or harass an individual, group, or organization.

It may include false accusations, defamation, slander and libel. It may also include monitoring, identity theft, threats, vandalism, solicitation for sex, or gathering information that may be used to threaten, embarrass or harass.

Cyberstalking is often accompanied by real time, offline stalking. In many jurisdictions, such as California, both are criminal offenses. Both are motivated by a desire to control, intimidate or influence a victim, according to the website.

A stalker may be an online stranger or a person whom the target knows. He may be anonymous and solicit involvement of other people online who do not even know the target.

Cyberstalking is a criminal offense under various state anti-stalking, slander and harassment laws.

A conviction can result in a restraining order, probation, or criminal penalties against the assailant, including jail.

The website, norton.us.com, also warns of Catfishing.

Catfishing is another method of online stalking. It's where the user poses as someone else, using social media sites.

They tend to use fake names, photos, and locations. They will often approach the victim as a love interest or a mutual friend.

Oftentimes, they will copy the profiles of an existing user as a way to verify their identity of a real person, the website says.

The Norton website lists ways to spot a fake profile:

>Do a reverse Google image search of the user's profile picture. If they're a fake, it will lead to you to multiple profiles or to a website that the catfisher pulled the image from.

Check how many friends the user's profile has. An average Facebook profile has about 130 friends. Catfishing profiles will have significantly less.

Examine the user's photos carefully. A real person will have photos of themselves with friends and family or at public events. Catfishers generally have selfies or modeling shots. Also, check to see if the other people in their photos are tagged, verifying that they are friends with the people in the photos.

If you suspect you're being catfished, ask the user to Skype via webcam to verify their identity. If they make up excuses, that is an indication of a red flag.

The website also provides these anti-stalking tips:

Maintain vigilance over physical access to your computer and other Web-enabled devices like cell phones. Cyberstalkers use software and hardware devices (sometimes attached to the back of your PC without you even knowing) to monitor their victims.

Be sure you always log out of your computer programs when you step away from the computer and use a screensaver with a password. The same goes for passwords on cell phones. Your kids and your spouse should develop the same good habits.

Make sure to practice good password management (link to password article) and security. Never share your passwords with others. And be sure to change your passwords frequently! This is very important.

Delete or make private any online calendars or itineraries — even on your social network — where you list events you plan to attend. They could let a stalker know where you're planning to be and when.

A lot of personal information is displayed on social networks, such as your name, date of birth, where you work and where you live. Use the privacy settings in all your online accounts to limit your online sharing with those outside your trusted circle. You can use these settings to opt out of having your profile appear when someone searches for your name. You can block people from seeing your posts and photos, too.

If you post photos online via social networks or other methods, be sure to turn off the metadata in the photo. The metadata reveals a lot of information about the photo, where and when it was taken, what device it was taken on and other private information.

Metadata comes from photos taken on a mobile phone, You can turn this off, usually a feature called geotagging, in your phone's settings. Use a security software program such as Norton Security to prevent spyware from being installed onto your computer via a phishing attack or an infected Web page.

Security software could allow you to detect spyware on your device and decrease your chances of being stalked.

The website also reminds you to change all of your online passwords if you break off a relationship. Even if you think that your ex-partner may not know them, you never really can be sure.

Be aware of your own online presence.

It's a good idea to check your "Googleability."

How much information can be found out about you online?

Have you ever Googled yourself? If not, you should, just so you can be aware of what personal information is out there about you.

Try different combinations, starting with just your full name. Then try your name plus your phone number, your name plus your home address and your name and your birthdate.

You can also search for your family members to see what is available about you through their profiles. If you happen to find that that there is sensitive personal information easily available, there are a few ways you can get it removed from the Internet.

In most cases, if it is a photo, or a website has information such as your address, telephone number or date of birth, contact the website and ask them to remove the data.

If it is sensitive personal information such as your Social Security number, bank account or credit card number, contact Google and they will remove it.

Finally, if you encounter a stalker and it seems serious, or you begin to receive threats, you should report it to the police.

Keep a copy of any message or online image that could serve as proof of cyberstalking.

Use the "print screen" or other keyboard functions to save screenshots. Many police departments have cybercrime units, and cyberstalking is a crime.

Cyberstalking is a form of cyberbullying, according to Sameer Hinduja of the website cyberbullying.org.

Hinduja defines cyberstalking as "willful and repeated harm inflicted through the use of computers, cell phones, and other electronic devices".

Cyberstalking behaviors may include tracking down someone's personal and private information and using it to make them afraid, texting them hundreds of times a day to let them know you are watching them, "creeping" on their social media accounts to learn where they are so you can show up there uninvited, or posting about them incessantly and without their permission.

"The common denominator is that the behavior makes the target extremely concerned for their personal safety and causes some form of distress, fear, or annoyance," Hinduja writes.

The National Center for Victims of Crime says it is important to trust your instincts. If you believe you have a stalker, take it seriously and contact law enforcement.

Stalkers are dangerous and have unpredictable behaviors, said Elaina Roberts, director of Strategic Initiatives at the victims of crime center told USA Today in 2018.

"Generally, when a person is being stalked, they often don't know where their stalker will be or what they will do," said Roberts.

Also, online stalking, or cyberstalking, should be taken seriously because it can spill over into the physical world, Roberts said.

CHAPTER ELEVEN

Create a safety plan

The National Center for Victims of Crime suggests creating a safety plan with a professional in order to prevent harm.

The plan can include a list of safe places, buying another phone that has a number only given out to trusted people, and varying your routine.

Tell your community.

"Relying on trusted friends and family is important for victims of stalking to help keep victims safer and also reduce the isolation and feelings of desperation that stalking victims may experience," stated the organization.

The organization suggests telling security guards, friends at work and school, giving copies of protective orders to schools or day-care centers, and talking with your children.

Document everything.

The National Center for Victims of Crime recommends keeping track of all the times a stalker has made contact, as well as when law enforcement was involved.
"Having the stalking log or protection order to show law enforcement will aid the officer in seeing the pattern of

behavior or course of conduct which criminal stalking statutes require," Roberts said.

Documents like photographs, text messages, emails, letters and time logs can help law enforcement.

Don't communicate with the stalker.

According to the National Center for Victims of Crime, 46 percent of stalking victims receive at least one unwanted contact per week.

"Stalkers are extremely persistent and have a high recidivism rate," Roberts said. "They usually don't stop the behavior even when victims communicate a desire for the behavior to stop. Any communication with the stalker can be taken as incentive to continue the behavior because the victim is paying attention to them."

A victim may choose to communicate with the stalker, though it's not recommended.

Roberts said some victims feel safer texting their stalker to discuss child custody or support payments.

CONCLUSION

Ultimately, you are responsible for your own safety.

While I titled this book "Heads Up! Self-defense for Journalists," obviously the information within this book is applicable to everyone, no matter what their profession.

I wrote the book for my fellow journalists because of the caustic atmosphere being perpetrated by President Donald Trump and his hateful and stupid "the media is the enemy of the people" rhetoric.

Here are a few final pointers.

If you can, I recommend you exercise regularly and become as fit as possible, as well as take some self-defense training.

Krav Maga is probably the best course for common sense, everyday self-defense. Brazilian Jujitsu is roundly considered a good self-defense art, but it — like karate and taekwondo — has a strong sportive aspect that can be dangerous. The traditional martial arts are effective, but take a long time for practitioners to truly become deadly. Krav Maga is more no-nonsense self-defense. Just be sure your instructor is certified through a legitimate organization — do a little research. Some fitness centers and strip-mall taekwondo schools teach a watered down version of Krav Maga that is more akin to fitness kickboxing than actual fighting.

Keep up with what is going on in your area, and use caution both meeting strangers (for example, while interviewing sources) and be retrospect in your social media use.

Look at your office, and see where security may be lax. Look for your own escape route in case of an active shooter event. Also load your desk with incidental weapons such as letter openers, scissors, and maybe even put a stout wooden cane or a baseball bat in the corner or under your desk.

Obviously, if you are licensed to conceal carry and you always have your gun with you, you may think the incidental weapons idea is superfluous, but it's always best to be prepared.

The same precautions should also taken in your automobile.

For good information on common sense self-defense, read:

"Defensive Living: When Defensive Driving, Diets, and Exercise Aren't Enough to Keep You Alive and Well!" by Bo Hardy.

Good luck, and stay safe!

www.ingramcontent.com/pod-product-compliance
Lightning Source LLC
Chambersburg PA
CBHW031258280526
45784CB00004B/1901